HIIT

What It Is and Why It Works

By PROSENCE

Respective authors own all copyrights not held by the publisher.

The information herein is offered for informational purposes solely, and is universal as so. The presentation of the information is without contract or any type of guarantee assurance.

The trademarks that are used are without any consent, and the publication of the trademark is without permission or backing by the trademark owner. All trademarks and brands within this book are for clarifying purposes only and are the owned by the owners themselves, not affiliated with this document.

ABOUT PROSENCE

Our Mission

We are dedicated to guiding, motivating and providing the tools necessary to transform people into the best version of themselves. Our goal is to empower men and women across the globe to realize that physical and mental fitness are not a short-term solution, but a lifetime choice, and to actualize what they have come to understand into a daily routine. We invite you to discover this process for yourself as you join us in the exploration of science-based knowledge that can lead to better health, greater fulfillment and astonishing vitality.

Who is Prosence?

Hi, I'm Antonio Mazzotta - certified Fitness Trainer and health enthusiast, and the founder of Prosence. While I don't think I'll ever turn down mom's homemade pasta and pizza, as an Italian living in Switzerland I've built a life dedicated to health and fitness. Now, I want to share the secrets to my success with you.

I got involved in this industry over 7 years ago, and quickly developed a passion for all things health and fitness. I knew right away that this is what I was born to do and haven't looked back. My days are spent developing new routines, training hard and meeting other fitness-minded and health-conscious individuals. I love working with my clients and coaching about weight training, dieting and healthy lifestyle choices. My number one priority is motivating people to achieve any fitness goal they seek. Whether you're looking to lose weight, get stronger, build cardio and endurance or just maintain overall health and vitality - I'm here to get you to your goals.

My team and I work hard to dispel the health and fitness myths and misinformation clogging the Internet today. We're driven by the desire to offer you a safe and manageable yet powerfully effective path to the best health of your life. Prosence is firmly committed to motivating, inspiring, and educating through the sharing of objective, fact-based health and fitness information that is rooted in science. We give you the tools you need to get in great shape and build a lifetime of good health.

Join us - let's work together to maximize your potential and achieve your optimal self while embracing life to the fullest!

Learn more on our website: www.prosencefitness.com, blog and keep up with the daily education and motivation by liking us on Twitter, Facebook & Instagram @prosencefitness.

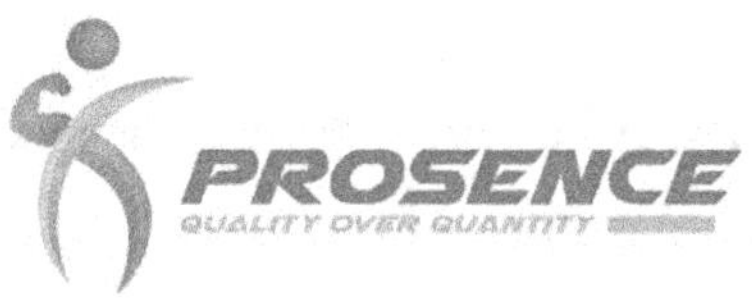

Table of Contents

Introduction

Many people have tried to achieve the body they've always dreamed of and the strength and fitness levels that go with it. While many have succeeded, much more have failed. And for those who have succeeded, they discovered one secret weapon that makes it much more possible to achieve their dream bodies and fitness levels - HIIT or High Intensity Interval Training.

Within this book's pages, you'll discover what HIIT really is, what are its foundational principles, what makes for the best HIIT workouts, and sample workouts to start you off HIITting. But beware though – once you're done reading this book, you may no longer have any excuses for not having your dream body and fitness and strength levels.

So if you're ready to start chiseling the body you want, turn the page and let's begin.

Chapter 1
What Is High Intensity Interval Training?

Many people think that eating's the only key to losing weight and getting in shape. While it's true that a big chunk of that's nutrition, physical training or exercise is equally important. And if you want to become really fit and athletic, all the more physical training becomes non-negotiable.

But physical training by any other type isn't necessarily as effective in helping you achieve your dream body and fitness level. Some will be much more effective while others hardly work. It all depends on your goals. If you want to be as muscular and bulky like Dwayne "The Rock" Johnson, a very heavy weight-lifting program's what the doctor will order. If you're after excellent cardiovascular conditioning, regular morning runs or brisk walks may be the most ideal types of training programs. But if you're looking to be lean and muscular – just like Ryan Reynolds or Zac Efron – and not like Ninja Turtle on steroids, then HIIT should be your workout of choice.

What is HIIT? It's a physical training program where you'll have to alternate high intensity exercises with a quicker period of low intensity exercises or rest. A very practical illustration is sprinting it with all you got for 20 seconds and resting completely for 10 seconds or another 20 seconds of a much lower intensity exercise like brisk walking for several cycles. Many people who've done HIIT programs will tell you that even if you do it for just 20 minutes 3 times a week, it can help burn more calories than brisk walking for 1 or 2 hours. That's how efficient and effective it is.

Phases

Practically speaking, you won't be able to sustain maximum physical effort while exercising for a long period of time. It's just not possible. And the reason what that's so is because your body was created to use calories in a different way. To help you get this better, let's assume that you try to sprint at all out effort for at least 20 minutes. Your body will go through several HIIT phases, such as:

– Phosphocreatine: While sprinting for the first 10 or 20 seconds, chances are you'll still feel great – excellent even! You'll probably think of yourself as an Maserati speeding down the freeway even if you look more like a speeding bicycle on a sidewalk. And why is that? It's because at the earliest part of your all out sprint, your muscles are still using its phosphocreatine reserves for high intensity energy.

- Anaerobic Glycolysis: After that short window of Euphoria, your muscles would've spent much if not all of its phosphocreatine reserves. At this point, lactic acid becomes the fuel of choice in lieu of phosphocreatine. When this happens, your body will continue feeling as if you're performing at top speed while in fact, you're running much slower than you think you are. Also, your lungs will start to feel like it's working extremely hard. So unless you're a freak of nature of an athlete like LeBron James, you probably won't be able to sustain this all out effort for 10 minutes. And if you're an average or below-average athlete, you'd probably have to stop running and catch your breath. But if you're a couch potato, it's possible that you may even throw up when you first do HIIT because of the sudden change in blood acidity levels.

If we were to simplify these things, we can say that the reason why you won't be able to go all out effort when you exercise for extended periods of time is oxygen. Yes, it's that all-essential element, particularly the body's demand for and the supply of such whenever you go all out physically. When you apply maximum intensity during physical activities, your body demands so much more oxygen compared to what is normally available. Hence, you can only choose between efficiency and intensity during physical activity, i.e., choosing efficiency (exercising longer) leads to lower intensity and vice versa.

When you choose to exercise at a relatively low intensity such as when going for a regular walk around the block, your body uses aerobic metabolism to utilize energy. Aerobic metabolism refers to how your body primarily uses carbohydrates and dietary fat for energy by using oxygen. This type of energy production process, a.k.a. metabolism, is great for endurance activities like running a half or full marathon but it's not so great for high intensity activities like swimming and running competitions.

And speaking of high intensity exercises that require max or almost max effort, a different type of metabolism takes effect: anaerobic. Remember how high intensity exercises lead your body to demand so much more oxygen than what's normally available? When your body lacks oxygen, it compensates by producing lactic acid as fuel. The challenge with lactic acid as a source of energy is that it's usually short-lived. It's a matter of time before you feel tired and unable to continue.

HIIT workouts allow you to marry these two seemingly incompatible partners to help you achieve your fitness goals. HIIT makes you alternate between aerobic and anaerobic metabolism, i.e., relatively longer periods of low intensity exercises like walking or total rest with high intensity exercises. You create a huge metabolic demand when you do short intervals of high intensity exercises, which can be a very effective way to shred stubborn body fat en route to higher fitness and conditioning levels. And when you shift to low or no intensity periods immediately after each high intensity interval, you give your body the chance to change to aerobic metabolism, which can let you recover enough energy quickly to do several rounds or intervals more of high intensity exercises.

Hormones

These are another group of crucial HIIT components. With low or no intensity activities like yoga or tai chi, stress hormones levels are low, which is a very good thing under normal circumstances. But considering your fitness and conditioning goals, low stress levels are undesirable. You'll need to increase your stress hormone levels, albeit for short periods of time only.

A primary measure of cardiovascular effort and fitness is the VO2 max, which is a measure of the maximum rate of oxygen consumption during exercise. HIIT workouts can raise your VO2 max levels to as high as 90%! At such high levels, your body secretes higher than usual levels of epinephrine, norepinephrine, cortisol, and aldosterone – all stress hormones. As a response to elevate stress hormone levels, your body secretes more testosterone and growth hormones, which are key elements to building optimal conditioning, fat burning, and muscle building. So for a brief period of time, elevated stress hormones help you change your body's composition (fat and lean body mass levels) and improve physical conditioning.

Essential HIITs

As is obvious by the name, HIIT exercises or routines are very intense naturally. Hence, they can lead to high stress hormone production. As you perform them, you put your body in a crisis state, where oxygen supply is way less than demand, your body temperature soars, body fluids and energy stores are depleted substantially, and tissues are damaged. And as a protective reaction, your body will create or produce higher levels of endocrine, which is things like low blood oxygen levels, acidosis, high carbon dioxide levels, elevated body temperature, dehydration, psychological stress, and physical injuries can do to your body.

Simply put, your body will "freak out" when you do HIIT. And as it does, your body will be forced to bring out its most effective weapons for defense. Because of the unusually high level of stress that high intensity physical activities can exercise on your body, it eventually force-activates its survival mechanism to adapt to higher and higher stress levels. As it does, it becomes more fit and conditioned.

Chapter 2
Why Bother With HIIT? Science And Evidence-Based Results

While it may seem that HIIT is counterproductive to your fitness and conditioning goals due to its ability to seriously stress your body out, even if for brief time periods only, it actually does provide substantial physical benefits such as:

- Ability to perform high intensity activities for longer time periods;

- Faster fat loss with minimal muscle wastage;

- Higher fast-twitch muscle fiber activation, which is crucial for top strength, power, and fitness;

- Higher tolerance for discomfort, perseverance, and resiliency (mental toughness);

- Significant cardiovascular fitness and health improvements; and

- Sports-centered energy systems that are more efficient and
  effective.

Lastly, you can have your cake and eat it too with HIIT. How?
You can achieve your dream body and conditioning within a
shorter period of time compared to most exercise routines?
How's 5 to 10 minute exercise or workout sessions sound to you
compared to more than 30 minutes of brisk walking or jogging?
Talk about more (fat burning) for less (time)!

Chapter 3
The Best HIIT Workouts

HITT workouts can be performed in a myriad number of ways through a wide range of exercise combinations. As such, there is really no single best HIIT workout, i.e., combination of exercises. But regardless of the workout or combination you choose, it can be the best HIIT workout for you if you perform any workout or exercise combination using specific durations for the intervals. And one such way of performing HIIT is the Tabata protocol.

The Tabata protocol is the most popular HIIT protocol today, which is 20 seconds of high intensity work followed by 10 seconds of low intensity exercise. The protocol came about as a result of a formal study called – you guessed it – the Tabata Study! During the study, the subjects were instructed to row at top speed for 20 seconds followed by 10 seconds of rowing at a relaxed pace, which was repeated for 8 cycles for a total of 4 minutes. Researchers discovered a 28% average increase in the participants' average anaerobic capacity and an average increase in VO2 max of about 14%.

Resistance Exercises And HIIT

Another characteristic of a "best" or optimal HIIT workout is working against a resistance or weight, i.e., resistance or weight lifting exercises. The kind of weight used doesn't matter – bodyweight or weights – for as long as it's a weight that you can perform the optimal number of repetitions with. Also, it's important that you perform multi-joint or compound exercises, which are exercises that involve multiple muscle groups like pull ups, push ups, and barbell squats, among others. Compound HIIT exercises are often referred to as oxygen suckers in that they can really make you feel like all the oxygen supply in the world has been used up.

It's inevitable that your body will reach a point where it has completely adjusted to the stress level you consistently subject it to with your HIIT workouts, in which case progress will plateau. In such cases, all you need to do is "re-stress" your body by simply changing the exercises or if you're using weights, increase the weights or resistance you're working with on the exercises. Doing so will put more stress on your body that it'll need to start adjusting to again and restart your progress in terms of achieving your dream body and conditioning levels.

Customized HIITs

Aside from the relatively shorter workout periods, another big advantage to doing HIIT workouts is the ease at which you can tailor fit or customize your workouts. What makes it possible is HIIT's very simple foundation: just alternate high intensity exercises with low intensity ones or with complete rest for several cycles or intervals. That's it. It's like your wardrobe that you can mix and match. In fact, you neither need to be a certified trainer nor need to be supervised by one if you want to perform HIIT and enjoy its benefits. However, it's still highly advisable to enlist the services of a trained professional when you start to do HIIT because through that professional, your chances of performing the exercises correctly and develop the right foundations are much higher compared to going Lone Ranger. But just the same, the lack of a certified fitness professional is not a hindrance for doing HIIT workouts and enjoying its benefits.

Customizing your HIITs doesn't just mean being able to change the exercises and their pecking order during your workouts. You can also tinker with the high and low intensity intervals' durations. The Tabata protocol may be the most popular way of doing HIIT but it doesn't mean you can't benefit by changing the duration of your high and low intensity exercises for your optimal benefit. It's important to realize that while some things fit most people, it doesn't necessarily fit all. It's the same with the Tabata protocol – it works for many people but it may not necessarily be the best for you. Or it may be such that because of your body's ability to adapt, it may be optimal at first and later on its efficacy declines as your body gets used to the stress it provides.

That being said, you can change the duration as you deem fit to ensure that your body never gets used to the stress level of your HIIT workouts and continue progressing towards your goals. You can do that by extending the high intensity duration, shortening the low or no intensity duration, or doing both. Just don't overdo it by going for more than 1 minute for either intervals. Too much effort can lead to burnout and too much rest can lead to under stimulation and render your workouts useless.

As a beginner, it's much better to err on the side of caution by doing shorter high intensity intervals and longer low intensity ones. As you get used to HIIT and your body adjusts accordingly, you can start upping up the ante.

Lower Risks For Injuries

But wait...there's more! Your risks for injuries are also much lower with HIIT. Why? Because you can change things up and customize your workouts, you minimize the risk of training your muscles and joints too much or forcing yourself to perform specific exercises that aren't quite compatible with your physiology. More importantly, you reduce your risks for a different kind of injury that afflicts most exercise newbies and causes them to quit – boredom! The option to mix and match keeps things fresh most of the time so that you don't get bored.

Intensity

One of the most common mistakes people who train make is to think that intensity is standard across everybody, i.e., intensity levels are the same for everybody. Be different and believe differently. Why?

The truth is that intensity levels vary according to each individual. For example, it's fairly low intensity for me to bench press a 60-pound barbell but for a petite person who has never exercised before, even 30 pounds is already high intensity. Therefore, intensity levels are subjective.

There are a lot of techniques to very accurately determine your workouts' intensity levels but many of them are very technical and complex. But there's a very simple but relatively accurate way of determining your intensity level – the Talk Test.

The talk test involves trying to talk while performing your workouts. If you can talk normally like you're not doing anything, then you're exercising at a low or even no intensity. If you're still able to carry a conversation albeit with some strain, you're exercising at mid-level intensity. If you can hardly carry a conversation, now that's high intensity. It's that simple.

What if you determine that your intensity level isn't up to par? You can increase the intensity two ways: speed and resistance. For speed, you can simply increase the rate at which you perform the movements, e.g., increase the number of repetitions per interval. For resistance, you can increase the weight or resistance your working against while performing the same number of reps for one interval.

Warming Up

When you exercise at the very high intensity, such as when doing high intensity interval trainings, it is crucial that you warm up properly. Doing so will help you minimize your risks forgetting injured, i.e., pulling a muscle, tearing a ligament, or getting lightheaded because of abruptly starting to exercise. There are two main stretches if you can do in terms of loosening up and warming your muscles: Static stretches and dynamic stretches. Static stretching involves holding a specific stretching position for a specific of time. But when it comes to high intensity interval training or HIIT, static stretches aren't beneficial. In fact, they can even be detrimental or harmful. This is because static stretches for your muscles to stretch as far as they can without the benefit of being warmed up or limbered up first. That's why when it comes to HIIT training warm ups, you must focus on doing dynamic stretches.

Dynamic stretches are those that require you to move your body as a means of loosening up your muscles and warming them up as well. These include brisk walking, jogging, bodyweight squats, torso twists, arm circles. Warming up to this way allows you to gradually loosen and warm up your muscles and thus, minimize your risks for lightheadedness or injuries.

Chapter 4
HIIT In Group Training

While HIIT is something you can perform or do on your own, training with a group or a class can help you achieve your goals better, faster, and with potentially much more results. There are several reasons for it.

First is training with a group regularly puts you in position of having to be accountable to not just one person but to several. Accountability is that sense of being answerable to someone if you're not able to do what you're supposed to do. When you join a group, there is some "peer pressure" to at least do the basics and do them to the best of your abilities, such as showing up for each and every training session and doing the prescribed exercises. You won't get that from training alone.

The second reason why HIIT in a group setting can work well for you is motivation. Training by yourself, especially with a relatively challenging workout such as HIIT can be very taxing on one's willpower and motivation. The temptation to slack off or stop altogether is quite strong in isolation. When you join

HIIT group classes, you can feed off the encouragement and motivation of other people in the group much like a piece of coal continues to burn when with many other pieces of burning coal. The flame of your HIIT passion can continue to burn strong when you train regularly with a group.

The third reason for joining a group for regular HIIT is personalized training. You may be thinking how dare I say that when by its very nature, group training isn't individualized. Here's the thing. When you train with a group, especially with one that is led by an instructor, you have the opportunity to be supervised by that instructor. While group instructors do train several people simultaneously, they can go around while the group performs the prescribed exercises to check who among the group isn't doing well, which includes you. Instructors can go to you and correct your form or tell you to either speed things up or slow things down, depending on your current fitness level. You can also adapt the group's training program as your own without having to hire your own personal trainer. That's a relatively cheap way of getting personal training, don't you think?

The last reason why group HIIT can work wonders for you is variety. With an able instructor supervising the group, the exercises, the durations, and combinations of both can be changed and mixed up in order to prevent your body from fully adapting to the stimulation that causes beneficial changes in your body's composition and conditioning. As part of a group, you won't have to concern yourself with having to ensure variety in your workouts.

Chapter 5
Sample Workouts

As we near the end of this book and having learned why HIIT works and how it works, it's time to hit the ground running. In this chapter, I'll show you 3 sample HIIT workouts you can start with. These are by no means hard and fast rules but are merely guides to help you see in practical terms how HIIT workouts look like.

Regardless of the workout you choose to perform, always begin with a 2-minute dynamic warm-up to loosen and prime up your muscles so that they'd be all good to go. You can do this by:

—   Marching or jogging in place for up to half a minute;

—   Perform "back strokes" by standing straight, and alternately moving each arm in a reverse circle for another half minute; and

—   Do front, side, and back lunges with the same leg for half a minute before doing the same with the other for another half minute.

Now, your body's all loose and warmed up to HIIT your workout!

The 10-Minute Version

With this simple routine, you can get a very good workout in less time than it takes you to even just go to the gym! And best of all, no equipment needed! Perform this routine 3 times, doing as many reps as you can for 20 seconds for each exercise, with each exercise followed by a 10 second rest period prior to the next exercise.

Here are the exercises:

- Boxer Moves: Begin by standing straight with your left foot in front of the right. Let your hips face the right side and assume a boxer's position, i.e., arms bent at a 90-degree angle at the elbows and raised up with your forearms perpendicular to the floor and upper arms parallel to the ground. Quickly punch forward with your left arm followed by a cross punch with your right arm. As you punch with the right arm, let your torso rotate at the waist. As you perform this, remember to keep your bodyweight on your left foot and allow your right foot's heel to slightly lift off the ground with the right forefoot still planted on the ground. Return to the original position and perform as many sets as you can for 20 seconds before resting for 10 seconds and doing the same facing the other side, i.e., right foot in front of the left and hips facing to the left side.

– Jumping Jacks: Stand straight with both feed as wide as your hips. Let your arms fall at the sides. Jump and let your feet spread outward as you land and as you do so, raise your arms to the side and over your head. Jump again and let your feet come together again at about hip width, letting your arms reverse the motion and return to the starting position. Repeat as many times as possible for 20 seconds, rest for 10 seconds, then repeat for 2 more times, with each followed by a 10-second rest.

– Japanese Squats: Spread your feet a bit wider than the width of your hips, with your toes pointing outward forming a 45-degree angle. Put your weight on your heels, lift your chest upright, keep your lower back straight, and bring your body down by squatting just until your thighs become parallel to the ground. Push your self back up to starting position and do as many reps as you can for 20 seconds, followed by a 10-second rest. Do this 3 times with a 10-second rest right after each set.

End the workout by cooling down with a forward fold, reverse lunges, and an overhead stretch.

The 20-Minute Version

For this higher intensity workout, you'll do 3 rounds where each exercise lasts for 45 seconds, followed by a 15-second rest. For each exercise, do as many repetitions as you can within the 45-second work period.

- Push Ups: If regular pushups are impossible for you given your current physical fitness and conditioning levels, you can perform these with your knees resting on the floor or your hands on a sturdy table or counter.

- Japanese Squats;

- Glute Kicks: While jogging or running in place, try to kick your butt with the heel of your elevated foot or leg.

- Triceps Dips: With your back to a chair, put both hands on a sturdy low table or bench/chair. Extend your legs out in front of you. Bending only at your elbows, gradually lower your body as low as you can to the ground before pushing yourself back up to the starting position. Remember to keep your core muscles tensed and tight throughout the whole movement for added workout.

- Lunges To The Side: Stand with your feet pointing straight ahead and your bodyweight on your heels. Take a wide step to the right side and perform a deep lateral or side lunge. Return to the starting position and alternate with the other leg/foot. Don't let your knees go past your toes while doing this movement to minimize risks for knee injuries.

End the workout with a quad stretch, a forward fold, and overhead stretch.

The 30-Minute Version

This half-hour version can give your core a very good challenge, in addition to being a great whole body workout. And what's more is that this routine can help you burn more calories – and body fat – than a 30-minute brisk walk on the treadmill or outdoors! You can warm up with the same dynamic warm up routine as the 2 shorter versions. Perform as many reps as you can for 45 seconds for each exercise followed by a 15-second rest period before moving to the next one. Perform 3 rounds.

– Push Ups;

– Japanese Squats;

– Glute Kicks;

– Triceps Dips;

– Lunges To The Side;

– Jumping Jacks; and

– Sit Ups.

For cooling down, you can do a forward fold, a reverse lunge, and a quad stretch with each one lasting for up to half a minute.

Chapter 6
FAQs

Do I Need Any Special Equipment For HIIT?

No you don't. You can choose to use equipment like barbells and dumbbells and other contraptions but if you don't have access to such equipment, you can get a very good HIIT workout using only your bodyweight. And if you noticed, the sample workouts in this book employ bodyweight exercises only. This is to make sure you can get your HIIT workouts in regardless of your location.

Why Does HIIT Involve Mostly Bodyweight Exercises?

It's because contrary to popular opinion, bodyweight exercises are actually more difficult to perform compared to those that use weights, particularly for people who don't lift heavy. One reason this is so is because bodyweight exercises normally require you to balance your self while performing them, which forces you to use more than just 1 muscle group. The more muscle groups you use in an exercise, the more calories you burn while performing it. And by using bodyweight exercises, you can no longer make excuses for why you're not able to exercise.

Do I Need To Be Home To Do HIIT?

Nope. Because you can do HIIT using only your bodyweight, you can pretty much do it anywhere you want to – at home, at the gym, or at your favorite park. Heck, you can even do it at the airport if you get bored waiting for your flight to board!

Are Tabata And HIIT Different?

No. As mentioned in an earlier chapter, Tabata or the Tabata Protocol is a way of performing HIIT and as such, it is HIIT.

Do I Need An Instructor To Do HIIT?

No, you don't. But I highly recommend hiring one if you can afford to do so, especially if you're a beginner. Doing so gives you the benefit of objective feedback regarding proper execution of exercises, which is key to minimizing risks for exercise related injuries.

Conclusion

I hope that through this, you've learned enough about HIIT – particularly why and how it works – to be able to start doing HIIT and achieve your dream body and be achieve the highest level of conditioning ever. But there's one thing that this book won't be able to give you – the impetus to actually start HIITing and achieve your physical and fitness goals. Only you can make yourself act on what you've learned here and apply them in order to achieve your goals. Knowing is only half the battle – the other half is applying what you know.

So get on your feet and start HIITing your fitness and conditioning goals. The best time to start your journey was neither yesterday nor tomorrow but today. Stop making excuses and depriving yourself of optimal fitness and conditioning already. It's time to get your dream body...now!

Thank you for purchasing this book, I hope you enjoyed it.

Finally, if you enjoyed this book then I'd like to ask you for a favor. Will you be kind enough to leave a review for this book on Amazon? It would be greatly appreciated!

Don't forget to follow us on Twitter, Facebook & Instagram and visit our website www.prosencefitness.com to get empowered, educated and inspired to become the best version of yourself in life! You deserve it.

www.ingramcontent.com/pod-product-compliance
Lightning Source LLC
Chambersburg PA
CBHW070749260726
48660CB00007B/3027